S0-AWQ-424

The
Exercise Log

A Personal Training Diary
for All Fitness Programs

Glenn Francis

A DELL TRADE PAPERBACK

A DELL TRADE PAPERBACK
Published by
Dell Publishing Co., Inc.
1 Dag Hammarskjold Plaza
New York, New York 10017

With special thanks to Cheryl Caplow and Lynn Sherlock.

Dell ® TM 681510, Dell Publishing Co., Inc.

ISBN: 0-440-52417-2

Printed in the United States of America

One Previous Edition

January 1987

10 9 8 7 6 5 4 3 2 1

FG

Contents

Introduction

Exercise is important. You've already accepted that. The benefits are enormous in improving the way you look and feel. You have invested in workout clothes and health club memberships. Now you ask, "Did anything change? Have I made any progress?" Without a positive, conclusive answer it is so easy to become discouraged. No wonder so many people quit their fitness programs.

Why do we give up, after working so hard?

The key to a successful workout program is measurable progress. Every inch you add or take off, every increase in strength and decrease in heart rate, reinforces your commitment to fitness.

The Exercise Log is your tool for setting goals and measuring achievements. It is a total exercise workbook you can use to record exercise workouts for six months. Detailed instructions, complete examples, and a clear, logical format will make this log the easiest part of your exercise program.

Glenn Francis

How to Use
The Exercise Log

First and Last Day Comparison Chart

Begin your log by filling in the *First and Last Day Comparison Chart*, using the First Day column. Start by recording the date, your height and weight. Weigh yourself on the same scale which you plan on using throughout the year (a good bathroom scale is fine). Next, fill in your resting pulse rate, percent of body fat, and pulse recovery rate (instructions for how to do these are on pages 12, 13 and 14). If you've had your blood pressure measured lately, enter that information also. Finally, take your body measurements with a tape measure and enter under Measurements (see page 18 for body measurement locations).

At the end of six months enter the same information from the *Six Month Summary* charts into the Last Day column. Add or subtract the numbers to determine your progress and enter this figure into the Gain/Loss column, placing an appropriate + or − sign.

Photos

Take a picture of yourself and attach it to the *Photo—First Day of the Log* page. It is most effective if the photos you take are full-length and wearing a bathing suit. Fill in your chest/bust, waist, and hips measurements in the indicated spaces. This will help you visualize the relationship of these numbers to your physical appearance.

Repeat every four weeks and attach to the *Photo* pages provided. At the end of the sixth month, attach the photo you take to the

How to Use
The Exercise Log

Photo—Last Day of the Log page (opposite the *First Day* page). You will then have a permanent, visual comparison of the results of your fitness program.

Weekly Log

Start each *Weekly Log* page by filling in your weight at the beginning of the week. Be sure to start each *Weekly Log* page on a Sunday, so each week throughout the year will always begin on Sunday and end on Saturday. At the end of four weeks you will be able to note entries in the *Four-Week Progress Chart*. Since the number of days vary in each month, the four *Weekly Log* charts will not always correspond exactly with calendar months. So don't try to match the beginning and endings of the *Weekly Log* and *Four-Week Progress Charts* with the beginning and endings of calendar months.

NAME OF EXERCISE

This column is used for entering the name of the exercises you perform. The first fifteen lines are designed to record strength training exercises. Simply enter the name or description of the exercise performed, such as *squats, bench press, arm curls, push-ups,* etc. The last five lines are designed to record your aerobic or endurance exercises. Enter the name of the exercise, such as *running, swimming, cycling,* or *aerobics* (aerobic dance).

The Exercise Log is not limited to either strength or aerobic training. Any form of exercise, stretching, or sport can be listed, and progress recorded under either heading.

How to Use
The Exercise Log

REPS
(Repetitions)

Many exercises are made up of sets of one movement repeated continuously, without stopping, for a specific number of times. These are called repetitions or *reps.*

Typical numbers of reps for exercises requiring weights are 8, 10, or 12. Many exercises rely only on your body weight for resistance. Examples are: *push-ups, dips, chin-ups*, and *sit-ups*. To determine the amount of reps for these exercises, do as many as possible so that the last few are very difficult to properly complete. Add resistance (weights) when the number of repetitions becomes excessive.

SETS

The Sets column is used to record the number of sets performed in a workout session. For example, do 10 bench presses continuously, then stop and rest. This is one *set* of ten *reps.* Now, do 10 more continuous bench presses and stop. This is the second *set.* Follow with 10 more bench presses and log entry is 3, (3 *sets* of 10 *reps*).

WT.
(Weight)

Use this column to record the amount of weight used during the performance of an exercise. To determine the proper amount of weight to use, start the exercise by performing 8 reps per set. Add enough weight so that the 9th rep is impossible to properly complete. When you are able to accomplish 12 reps, add more weight until you can only perform 8 reps. Continue making progress in this fashion. This method can also be applied to timed or measured exercises. Strive for that extra five minutes or quarter mile for each exercise.

Example:

NAME OF EXERCISE	SUN		
	REPS	SETS	WT.
1. Bench Presses	12	3	100

TIME OR DISTANCE

Use this column (under the *AEROBICS* heading) to record either the time spent or distance covered for your aerobic or endurance training. At the end of each week, you can add the columns together to obtain your total time or distance for each exercise.

Example:

AEROBICS	SUN TIME / DISTANCE
1. Running	5 mi.
2. Aerobic Dance	1 hr.

Notes and Comments

Use this space to comment on things like weather conditions, training partners, instruction or equipment performance. Also, there are factors which can affect your daily exercise program such as sleep, diet, and attitude. Keeping track of these factors will help you to make an overall evaluation of your exercise program.

How to Use
The Exercise Log

Four-Week Progress Chart

At the end of every fourth *Weekly Log* there appears a *Four-Week Progress Chart*. This chart enables you to summarize achievements, and provides an easy reference for review.

Begin by entering the dates covered and your body weight information. Next, list the exercises you performed during the last four weeks. Enter both the beginning and ending information for the month. Add or subtract the beginning and ending numbers to determine your monthly gain or loss for each exercise. Finally, add or subtract these numbers from the previous month to determine your progress from the first day.

In the *AEROBICS* section, fill in the total time or distance for each week from the *Weekly Log* pages. Add or subtract the four weekly totals together to determine your total for the month. Finally, add the monthly total to the previous monthly total to obtain your new total from the first day.

Goals for Next Month

Now that you've recorded the results of your exercises for the month, take a few minutes to review and analyze the figures. Based on this information, write down what you would like to accomplish. This is a good time to establish your goals for the following month.

Six Month Summaries

After the sixth *Four-Week Progress Chart* are three *Six Month Summary* charts, each designed to summarize different information. Simply list the exercises you performed under each category and record your progress at the end of each month.

How to Use
The Exercise Log

At the end of six months, either add or subtract the first and last month numbers to determine your progress from the first day. Enter your current weight and measurements in the proper charts.

Record this information in the *First and Last Day Comparison Chart* under the Last Day heading.

Based upon your accomplishments, plan your fitness goals for the next six months and write them on the *Goals for Next Six Months* pages provided.

The Exercise Log is your personal exercise workbook. As you move along from week to week, you will realize the significance of your log entries. You might also notice there were many details you left out. Each week, strive to record more and more details of your exercise experiences. At the end of six months you will find that *The Exercise Log* has become one of your most valuable workout tools.

Fitness Ratings

There are four common ways to measure your level of physical fitness. It is important to know your current level of fitness in order to set attainable fitness goals.

This section explains these methods of measurement. The charts provide an indication of your fitness level in each category. Use this information to define your goals and design your personal exercise program.

RESTING PULSE RATE

Your resting pulse (or heart) rate is the most simple and accurate method for measuring your level of physical fitness. A low resting pulse indicates a strong heart, and a high number of beats per minute can indicate a weak heart.

Measure your resting pulse rate first thing in the morning, while you are still in bed. Using your first two fingers, place them together on the inside of your wrist. Be sure that the palm is facing up and that you are feeling for the pulse on the side of the wrist directly below your thumb. Count the number of beats for one full minute. Compare your result with the chart below.

	MEN	WOMEN
EXCELLENT	Lower — 60	Lower — 64
GOOD	61 — 68	65 — 72
FAIR	69 — 75	73 — 79
POOR	76 — Higher	80 — Higher

Fitness Ratings

PERCENT OF BODY FAT

An excellent indication of your fitness level is your percent of body fat relative to lean muscle tissue. Muscle is heavier than fat and a scale cannot differentiate between them. This means that your body weight alone is not a good indication of your ideal weight. A more accurate method of measurement is the skin fold or pinch test.

You can perform a skin fold test yourself by simply pinching the skin on the back of your upper arm, midway between your shoulder and elbow. Pull the pinched area away from the muscle and measure the thickness of the fold with a ruler. For a man the measurement should be less than ¾ inches. For a woman, less than 1 inch. Anything more than 1 inch for a man or 1-1/2 inches for a woman usually indicates obesity. The basic rule of thumb is that if you can "pinch an inch" of fat anywhere on your body, then you need to reduce your body fat level.

Most fitness centers and physicans can accurately measure your body fat percentage by taking skinfolds from several areas and measuring them with calipers. If you have this information, then you can use it to compare with the chart below.

	MEN	WOMEN
EXCELLENT	Lower — 10%	Lower — 13%
GOOD	11% — 16%	14% — 19%
FAIR	17% — 23%	20% — 26%
POOR	24% — Higher	27% — Higher

Fitness Ratings

PULSE RECOVERY RATE

This test can help determine fitness by measuring the decrease in pulse rate after exercise has stopped.

To perform this test, you must exercise strenuously enough to elevate your pulse between 70 percent to 90 percent of your maximum heart rate (see chart on page 17). At this point take your pulse for six seconds then multiply by 10 to obtain your Exercise Pulse. Wait exactly 60 seconds (one minute) then take your pulse again for six seconds. Again multiply by 10. This is your One Minute Pulse. Subtract your One Minute Pulse (second number) from your Exercise Pulse (first number) to determine your Pulse Recovery Rate.

Formula:

$$\begin{array}{r} \text{Exercise Pulse} \\ - \quad \text{One Minute Pulse} \\ \hline = \quad \text{Pulse Recovery Rate} \end{array}$$

A high number (quick recovery) indicates a healthy heart. Compare your pulse recovery rate with the chart below.

EXCELLENT	60 — Higher
GOOD	40 — 50
FAIR	20 — 30
POOR	Lower — 10

BLOOD PRESSURE

Your blood pressure is an indicator of the condition of your arteries, cardiovascular system, and level of stress. High blood pressure can indicate restricted arteries, mental stress, or other cardiovascular disorders.

Blood pressure is measured by two numbers. The top number (systolic) is the pressure exerted when the heart pumps, and the bottom number (diastolic) indicates the pressure between heart beats.

Taking your blood pressure requires some specialized equipment. If you have the correct equipment available to you, then you can measure it yourself. However, most of us depend on our personal physician to take our blood pressure for us. If this is the case, ask your physician for this information each time you visit. Compare your blood pressure with the chart below.

	SYSTOLIC		DIASTOLIC
LOW	110	/	75
AVERAGE	120	/	80
HIGH	140	/	90
VERY HIGH	160	/	95

Height and Weight Tables

The following tables are an indication of desirable body weights, based on longevity. Keep in mind that this chart, like any other, is merely a comparison guide. Your personal body weight objective should be based on your percent of body fat.

MEN

HEIGHT		WEIGHT IN POUNDS		
FT.	IN.	SMALL FRAME	MEDIUM FRAME	LARGE FRAME
5	2	110 – 118	116 – 127	124 – 139
5	3	113 – 122	119 – 131	127 – 142
5	4	116 – 124	122 – 134	130 – 146
5	5	119 – 127	125 – 137	133 – 150
5	6	122 – 131	130 – 141	136 – 154
5	7	128 – 135	132 – 145	140 – 159
5	8	130 – 139	136 – 150	145 – 164
5	9	134 – 143	140 – 154	149 – 168
5	10	138 – 148	144 – 158	153 – 172
5	11	142 – 152	148 – 163	157 – 177
6	0	146 – 156	152 – 168	162 – 182
6	1	150 – 160	156 – 173	166 – 187
6	2	154 – 165	160 – 178	171 – 192
6	3	158 – 169	165 – 183	176 – 197
6	4	162 – 173	170 – 188	180 – 202

WOMEN

HEIGHT		WEIGHT IN POUNDS		
FT.	IN.	SMALL FRAME	MEDIUM FRAME	LARGE FRAME
4	10	90 – 96	94 – 105	102 – 117
4	11	92 – 99	96 – 108	104 – 120
5	0	94 – 102	99 – 111	107 – 123
5	1	97 – 105	102 – 114	110 – 126
5	2	100 – 108	105 – 117	113 – 129
5	3	103 – 111	108 – 120	116 – 132
5	4	106 – 114	111 – 124	119 – 136
5	5	109 – 117	114 – 128	123 – 140
5	6	112 – 121	118 – 133	127 – 144
5	7	116 – 125	122 – 137	131 – 148
5	8	120 – 129	126 – 141	135 – 152
5	9	124 – 133	130 – 145	139 – 156
5	10	128 – 138	134 – 149	143 – 161
5	11	132 – 142	138 – 153	147 – 166
6	0	136 – 146	142 – 157	151 – 171

Without shoes or clothing, over age 25. Metropolitan Life Insurance Co.

Target Heart Rate for Aerobic Exercise

In order to gain the maximum benefit from your aerobic workouts, you must increase your heart rate to at least 70 percent of your maximum and no more than 90 percent. This is the *target heart rate* or *training zone*. Only by exercising at this level will you be working the heart hard enough to increase its strength. The chart below graphically indicates the number of beats per minute, in relation to age, that your heart should be working during performance of aerobic exercise.

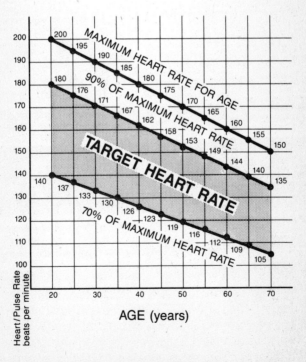

Formula for Maximum Heart Rate: 220 minus age.

Where to Take Body Measurements

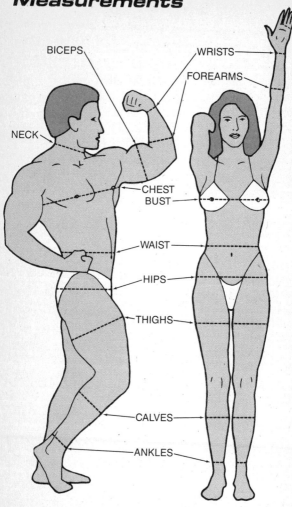

BICEPS

WRISTS

FOREARMS

NECK

CHEST
BUST

WAIST

HIPS

THIGHS

CALVES

ANKLES

Measurements should be taken before exercising. A "cold" measurement is more reliable then directly after a vigorous workout when your muscles are temporarily "pumped up." For chest or bust measurements, take a deep breath so that your chest is fully expanded.

First and Last Day Comparison Chart

From: (first day) ____ / ____ / ____ To: (last day) ____ / ____ / ____

	FIRST DAY	LAST DAY	GAIN/LOSS	
HEIGHT			+ OR −	
WEIGHT				
RESTING PULSE RATE				
PERCENT OF BODY FAT				
PULSE RECOVERY RATE				
BLOOD PRESSURE	——	——	—	——
Measurements				
CHEST / BUST				
WAIST				
HIPS				
NECK				
SHOULDERS				
RIGHT BICEPS				
LEFT BICEPS				
RIGHT FOREARM				
LEFT FOREARM				
WRISTS				
RIGHT THIGH				
LEFT THIGH				
RIGHT CALF				
LEFT CALF				
ANKLES				

Photo — First Day of Log

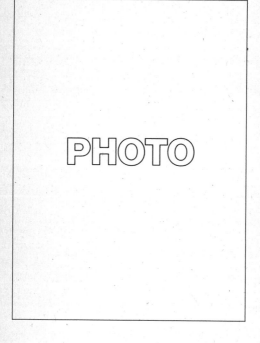

WEIGHT   _____

CHEST/BUST _____

WAIST   _____

HIPS   _____

Photo—Last Day of Log

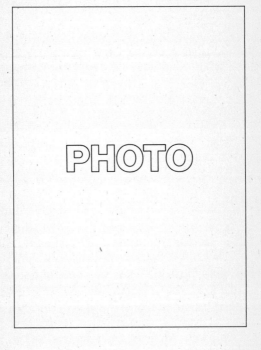

WEIGHT _____

CHEST/BUST _____

WAIST _____

HIPS _____

Exercise Training Tips

This section includes some methods and recommendations for anyone considering or already involved in an exercise program. They are intended to help you achieve the best possible results from your fitness program.

Physical Exam If you have had a fairly sedentary life-style and have not been exercising on a regular basis, consult your physican before beginning any exercise program. To suddenly exert abnormal stress on your heart and muscles can cause a variety of problems ranging from muscle strains to fatal heart attack. If you are over thirty years old, it is advisable that you complete a stress test (stress electrocardiogram or EKG).

Warm-Ups It is very important that you warm up your body and muscles before attempting any form of exercise. Suddenly plunging cold, tight muscles into vigorous activity can pull, strain, or otherwise injure muscles, tendons, and joints.

A good warm-up is needed to increase body and muscle temperature so that your muscles and connective tissues are supple and pliable. The best muscle warmer is your own circulation. The warm-ups will increase your heart rate and circulation, which will nourish your muscles with blood and oxygen.

Warm, nourished, supple muscles perform far better, thus enabling you to make greater athletic achievements.

Begin your warm-ups with light aerobic activity such as running in place to stimulate your respiratory and circulatory systems. Your objective is to gradually increase your body temperature and warm your muscles before going on to stretching.

Exercise Training Tips

You should spend from ten to fifteen minutes on warm-ups prior to stretching or exercising.

Stretching Once your internal temperature is raised by the warm-ups, you are ready to stretch your muscles to achieve greater flexibility, coordination, elasticity, and increased range of motion. This will enable you to give 100 percent intensity to your workouts.

The objective of stretching is to lengthen your muscles, tendons, and ligaments as much as possible. Stretching should be done both before exercising and after. Stretch before exercising in order to prepare for the transition to vigorous activity without undue strain, and to increase your muscles' range of motion. A longer range of motion will yield greater muscular development.

Stretching should also be done after exercising. The greatest gains in flexibility are made when stretching muscles that are very warm, such as directly after exercise. It is then that the muscle can really lengthen without risk of injury. Since it is warm and willing to be shaped, it can be stretched just a little bit more. If you only have time to stretch once, after the activity is the most beneficial.

The most important thing to remember about stretching is to slowly ease into the stretch and *not to bounce.* If a relaxed muscle is stretched too quickly, it can be easily torn. If you attempt to stretch your muscles too fast or too far, your body will automatically try to protect itself by contracting the stretched muscle. This protective mechanism is called the "stretch reflex." Bouncing stretches the muscle past its limit, thus tearing and injuring the muscle fiber. This is exactly the opposite of what you want to accomplish.

Exercise Training Tips

To properly stretch a muscle, slowly ease into the stretch to avoid triggering the stretch reflex. Your body should be relaxed. Concentrate on where the pulling sensation is. You should feel the pull in the meaty part throughout the bulk of the muscle. Stretching correctly feels good. It should not hurt or cause your muscles to feel sore or stiff afterwards.

Spend about five to ten minutes stretching before exercising, and about ten to twenty minutes after.

Cool-Downs   Just as you must prepare your body for exercise by warming up, a gradual cool-down period at the end of the workout is equally important.

During exercise your heart is pumping at an accelerated rate in order to respond to an increased demand for oxygenated blood by your muscles. If you suddenly stop exercising, your heart will continue to provide a high rate of blood flow, causing blood to "pool" in the muscles, especially in the legs. This can create a shortage of blood in the brain, resulting in dizziness or fainting. A gradual cool-down period can prevent this.

Cool-downs can also reduce the soreness or stiffness following a workout. This can help release the carbon dioxide and a toxin called lactic acid that accumulate during exercise to work their way out of your muscles.

Like the warm-ups, your cool-down period should last at least five minutes, to allow your heart a chance to adjust to its normal level. The cool-down activities are basically the same as the warm-ups, only in reverse. You are gradually decreasing your heart rate instead of increasing it.

Exercise Training Tips

Training Partners   It is best to train with a partner, both for safety in case you cannot complete a lift, and to assist each other with setting up and moving the weights. Training with a partner will make exercising more enjoyable and you will be less tempted to miss workouts.

Correct Level   Select your weight load so that you can perform between 8 to 12 repetitions. If you can do more, the weight is too light. Less than 6 reps is too heavy.

Form   Repetitions should be performed in a smooth and controlled manner. Apply a slow, steady force through the entire range of movement, from full extension to full flexion. Jerking or throwing the weights is counter-productive and can result in injury.

Breathing   When weight training, you should breathe normally and don't hold your breath. Holding your breath while lifting can be dangerous, since it raises your blood pressure and can cause you to pass out. There is no rule as to any particular breathing pattern, though usually people will exhale when exerting force and inhale at the beginning and ending of a lift.
   When exercising aerobically, you should not continue to exercise so hard that you cannot talk. If you cannot say out loud a short sentence or two, you should decrease your exertion.

Intensity   Continue each exercise until no additional repetitions are possible. This is called reaching the point of muscular failure or "training to failure." Maximum progress is made by putting 100 percent effort into each set. Intensity

Exercise Training Tips

can be increased by either adding resistance, performing more repetitions, or decreasing resting time between sets.

Interval Training   At the completion of a set of exercises, a rest period is needed in order for the muscles to recuperate. This is called the "rest interval" and usually lasts between one and two minutes before beginning the next set. Interval training for aerobic exercise consists of alternating between periods of intense and light workouts.

Frequency   After a workout, muscles need a recovery period of at least 48 hours but not more than 96 hours in order to grow. You should not work the same muscles every day. You can workout every day as long as you work different muscle groups.

Negative Repetitions   In addition to performing positive repetitions (the lifting half of a rep), you can also perform sets of negative repetitions (the lowering half of a rep). Add approximately 40 percent more weight than you normally use and go through your routine, performing 8 to 12 reps for each set. You will need a partner to help you lift the weight for each positive rep, and then you perform the lowering (negative) half unaided.

   You should also incorporate "negative accentuation" into all your workout routines. Simply take double the time to lower the weight than you take to raise it.

Machines   When training on exercise machines, you should begin to raise the weight at the point just before the weights touch the stack of remaining weights. Don't let the weights rest on the stack between reps.

It is also important to set the seat at the correct height. For rotary-cam machines such as Nautilus, the axis of the cam should be in line with the joint of the body part that is being worked. Remember to use the seat belts.

Free Weights   Always use collars to secure the weights (plates) to the barbell or dumbbells. Most weight training accidents are caused by weights falling off the bar.

Progression   Strive to increase the amount of weight or repetitions during every workout session. Only by subjecting your muscles to progressively greater and greater amounts of stress will they result in growth. Continuously working out with the same amount of weight will not increase strength. Be careful, however, not to sacrifice form in order to produce results.

Overtraining   Exercise is a good thing — but don't overdo it. Your muscles must be allowed adequate time to recover and grow before being stressed again. Working out too often, overly prolonging your workouts, or remaining with the same routine for too long can become non-productive, a condition referred to as overtraining. Symptoms include overly sore muscles, insomnia, loss of appetite, and apathy.

To cure overtraining, discontinue your workouts for one week, change your routine, reduce the number of sets, and increase intensity.

Weekly Log

Body Weight — Beginning of Week __187__   End of Week __188__   From: _1_ , _5_ , 86 To: _1_ , _11_ , 86   Gain/Loss (+ or –) _+1_ lb.

NAME OF EXERCISE	SUN REPS	SETS	WT.	MON REPS	SETS	WT.	TUE REPS	SETS	WT.	WED REPS	SETS	WT.	THU REPS	SETS	WT.	FRI REPS	SETS	WT.	SAT REPS	SETS
1. Bench Press				8	6	180				9	5	185				12	6	200		
2. Pull·Downs				10	4	230				10	4	240				12	6	240		
3. Arm Curls				8	3	100				10	4	100				10	6	100		
4. Seated Press				12	6	190				12	6	205				12	6	220		
5. Side Lateral Flies				10	4	55				12	5	60				12	6	70		
6. Pulley Rows				10	6	250				10	7	260				6	4	275		
7. Tricep Ext.				12	3	90				12	4	90				10	5	100		
8. Incline D.B. Flies				11	5	70				–	–	–				12	6	80		
9. Squats							12	8	380				14	6	400					

28

	SUN TIME/DISTANCE	MON TIME/DISTANCE	TUE TIME/DISTANCE	WED TIME/DISTANCE	THU TIME/DISTANCE	FRI TIME/DISTANCE	SAT TIME/DISTANCE	TOTAL FOR WEEK
10. Leg Press				8 6 490		6 6 510		
11. Leg Curls				12 5 120		12 6 130		
12. Thigh Extensions				13 4 200		12 5 220		
13. Hyper-extensions				25 3 25		— — —		
14. Sit-ups				60 4 —		70 4 —		
15. Toe Raises				15 3 450		10 5 460		
AEROBICS	SUN TIME/DISTANCE	MON TIME/DISTANCE	TUE TIME/DISTANCE	WED TIME/DISTANCE	THU TIME/DISTANCE	FRI TIME/DISTANCE	SAT TIME/DISTANCE	TOTAL FOR WEEK
1. Running	60 min./4½ mi.		60 min./5 mi.			70 min./6 mi.		3 hrs. 10 min./15½ mi.
2. Aerobic Dance		1 hr.					1 hr.	2 hrs.
3. Swimming	30 min./80 laps						45 min./100 laps	1 hr. 10 min./180 laps
4. Cycling					2½ hrs.			2½ hrs.
5. Stationary Bike				1½ hr.			1 hr.	2½ hrs.

Weekly Log

Body Weight — Beginning of Week _____ End of Week _____   From: ___ / ___ / ___   To: ___ / ___ / ___   Gain/Loss (+ or –) _____

NAME OF EXERCISE	SUN			MON			TUE			WED			THU			FRI			SAT		
	REPS	SETS	WT.	REPS	SETS	WT.	REPS	SETS	WT.	REPS	SETS	WT.	REPS	SETS	WT.	REPS	SETS	WT.	REPS	SETS	WT.
1.																					
2.																					
3.																					
4.																					
5.																					
6.																					
7.																					
8.																					
9.																					

AEROBICS

	SUN TIME / DISTANCE	MON TIME / DISTANCE	TUE TIME / DISTANCE	WED TIME / DISTANCE	THU TIME / DISTANCE	FRI TIME / DISTANCE	SAT TIME / DISTANCE	TOTAL FOR WEEK
1.								
2.								
3.								
4.								
5.								
10.								
11.								
12.								
13.								
14.								
15.								

Weekly Log

Body Weight — Beginning of Week _____ End of Week _____ From: ___/___/___ To: ___/___/___ Gain/Loss (+ or −) _____

NAME OF EXERCISE	SUN			MON			TUE			WED			THU			FRI			SAT		
	REPS	SETS	WT.	REPS	SETS	WT.	REPS	SETS	WT.	REPS	SETS	WT.	REPS	SETS	WT.	REPS	SETS	WT.	REPS	SETS	WT.
1.																					
2.																					
3.																					
4.																					
5.																					
6.																					
7.																					
8.																					
9.																					

AEROBICS	SUN TIME / DISTANCE	MON TIME / DISTANCE	TUE TIME / DISTANCE	WED TIME / DISTANCE	THU TIME / DISTANCE	FRI TIME / DISTANCE	SAT TIME / DISTANCE	TOTAL FOR WEEK
1.								
2.								
3.								
4.								
5.								
10.								
11.								
12.								
13.								
14.								
15.								

Weekly Log

From: ___ / ___ / ___ To: ___ / ___ / ___

Body Weight — Beginning of Week _____ End of Week _____ Gain/Loss (+ or −) _____

NAME OF EXERCISE	SUN			MON			TUE			WED			THU			FRI			SAT		
	REPS	SETS	WT.	REPS	SETS	WT.	REPS	SETS	WT.	REPS	SETS	WT.	REPS	SETS	WT.	REPS	SETS	WT.	REPS	SETS	WT.
1.																					
2.																					
3.																					
4.																					
5.																					
6.																					
7.																					
8.																					
9.																					

AEROBICS

	SUN TIME/DISTANCE	MON TIME/DISTANCE	TUE TIME/DISTANCE	WED TIME/DISTANCE	THU TIME/DISTANCE	FRI TIME/DISTANCE	SAT TIME/DISTANCE	TOTAL FOR WEEK
1.								
2.								
3.								
4.								
5.								
10.								
11.								
12.								
13.								
14.								
15.								

Weekly Log

From: ___ / ___ / ___   To: ___ / ___ / ___

Body Weight — Beginning of Week _____ End of Week _____ Gain/Loss (+ or −) _____

NAME OF EXERCISE	SUN			MON			TUE			WED			THU			FRI			SAT		
	REPS	SETS	WT.	REPS	SETS	WT.	REPS	SETS	WT.	REPS	SETS	WT.	REPS	SETS	WT.	REPS	SETS	WT.	REPS	SETS	WT.
1.																					
2.																					
3.																					
4.																					
5.																					
6.																					
7.																					
8.																					
9.																					

AEROBICS	SUN TIME / DISTANCE	MON TIME / DISTANCE	TUE TIME / DISTANCE	WED TIME / DISTANCE	THU TIME / DISTANCE	FRI TIME / DISTANCE	SAT TIME / DISTANCE	TOTAL FOR WEEK
1.								
2.								
3.								
4.								
5.								
10.								
11.								
12.								
13.								
14.								
15.								

Notes and Comments

Notes and Comments

Four-Week Progress Chart

Body Weight — Beginning of Month _____ End of Month _____ Gain/Loss (+ or –) _____

From: __ / __ / __ To: __ / __ / __

NAME OF EXERCISE	BEGINNING OF MONTH			END OF MONTH			GAIN/LOSS FOR MONTH				GAIN/LOSS FROM 1st DAY			
	REPS	SETS	WT.	REPS	SETS	WT.	+ OR –	REPS	+ OR –	SETS	+ OR –	WT.	+ OR –	REPS	+ OR –	SETS	+ OR –	WT.
1.														
2.														
3.														
4.														
5.														
6.														
7.														
8.														
9.														

PROGRESS 1

AEROBICS	TOTAL FOR WEEK #1	TOTAL FOR WEEK #2	TOTAL FOR WEEK #3	TOTAL FOR WEEK #4	TOTAL FOR THIS MONTH	FROM 1st DAY LAST MONTH	NEW TOTAL FROM 1st DAY
1.							
2.							
3.							
4.							
5.							
10.							
11.							
12.							
13.							
14.							
15.							

Photo

PHOTO

WEIGHT   _____
CHEST/BUST   _____
WAIST   _____
HIPS   _____

Goals For Next Month

_____
_____
_____
_____
_____
_____
_____
_____
_____
_____
_____
_____
_____
_____
_____
_____
_____
_____
_____
_____
_____
_____
_____
_____
_____
_____

Weekly Log

Body Weight — Beginning of Week _____ End of Week _____ Gain/Loss (+ or −) _____

From: ___ / ___ / ___   To: ___ / ___ / ___

NAME OF EXERCISE	SUN			MON			TUE			WED			THU			FRI			SAT		
	REPS	SETS	WT.	REPS	SETS	WT.	REPS	SETS	WT.	REPS	SETS	WT.	REPS	SETS	WT.	REPS	SETS	WT.	REPS	SETS	WT.
1.																					
2.																					
3.																					
4.																					
5.																					
6.																					
7.																					
8.																					
9.																					

AEROBICS	SUN TIME/DISTANCE	MON TIME/DISTANCE	TUE TIME/DISTANCE	WED TIME/DISTANCE	THU TIME/DISTANCE	FRI TIME/DISTANCE	SAT TIME/DISTANCE	TOTAL FOR WEEK
1.								
2.								
3.								
4.								
5.								
10.								
11.								
12.								
13.								
14.								
15.								

45

Weekly Log

Body Weight — Beginning of Week _____ End of Week _____ From: ___/___/___ To: ___/___/___ Gain/Loss (+ or −) _____

NAME OF EXERCISE	SUN			MON			TUE			WED			THU			FRI			SAT		
	REPS	SETS	WT.	REPS	SETS	WT.	REPS	SETS	WT.	REPS	SETS	WT.	REPS	SETS	WT.	REPS	SETS	WT.	REPS	SETS	WT.
1.																					
2.																					
3.																					
4.																					
5.																					
6.																					
7.																					
8.																					
9.																					

AEROBICS	SUN TIME / DISTANCE	MON TIME / DISTANCE	TUE TIME / DISTANCE	WED TIME / DISTANCE	THU TIME / DISTANCE	FRI TIME / DISTANCE	SAT TIME / DISTANCE	TOTAL FOR WEEK
1.								
2.								
3.								
4.								
5.								
10.								
11.								
12.								
13.								
14.								
15.								

Weekly Log

From: ___ / ___ / ___   To: ___ / ___ / ___

Body Weight — Beginning of Week _____ End of Week _____ Gain/Loss (+ or −) _____

NAME OF EXERCISE	SUN			MON			TUE			WED			THU			FRI			SAT		
	REPS	SETS	WT.	REPS	SETS	WT.	REPS	SETS	WT.	REPS	SETS	WT.	REPS	SETS	WT.	REPS	SETS	WT.	REPS	SETS	WT.
1.																					
2.																					
3.																					
4.																					
5.																					
6.																					
7.																					
8.																					
9.																					

AEROBICS	SUN TIME / DISTANCE	MON TIME / DISTANCE	TUE TIME / DISTANCE	WED TIME / DISTANCE	THU TIME / DISTANCE	FRI TIME / DISTANCE	SAT TIME / DISTANCE	TOTAL FOR WEEK
1.								
2.								
3.								
4.								
5.								
10.								
11.								
12.								
13.								
14.								
15.								

Weekly Log

Body Weight — Beginning of Week _____ End of Week _____

From: ___/___/___ To: ___/___/___

Gain/Loss (+ or −) _____

NAME OF EXERCISE	SUN			MON			TUE			WED			THU			FRI			SAT		
	REPS	SETS	WT.	REPS	SETS	WT.	REPS	SETS	WT.	REPS	SETS	WT.	REPS	SETS	WT.	REPS	SETS	WT.	REPS	SETS	WT.
1.																					
2.																					
3.																					
4.																					
5.																					
6.																					
7.																					
8.																					
9.																					

AEROBICS	SUN TIME / DISTANCE	MON TIME / DISTANCE	TUE TIME / DISTANCE	WED TIME / DISTANCE	THU TIME / DISTANCE	FRI TIME / DISTANCE	SAT TIME / DISTANCE	TOTAL FOR WEEK
1.								
2.								
3.								
4.								
5.								
10.								
11.								
12.								
13.								
14.								
15.								

Notes and Comments

Notes and Comments

Four-Week Progress Chart

Body Weight — Beginning of Month _____ End of Month _____ From: __/__/__ To: __/__/__ Gain/Loss (+ or –) _____

2 MONTHLY

NAME OF EXERCISE	BEGINNING OF MONTH			END OF MONTH			GAIN/LOSS FOR MONTH				GAIN/LOSS FROM 1st DAY			
	REPS	SETS	WT.	REPS	SETS	WT.	+ or –	REPS + or –	SETS + or –	WT.	+ or –	REPS + or –	SETS + or –	WT.
1.														
2.														
3.														
4.														
5.														
6.														
7.														
8.														
9.														

PROGRESS 2

AEROBICS

	TOTAL FOR WEEK #1	TOTAL FOR WEEK #2	TOTAL FOR WEEK #3	TOTAL FOR WEEK #4	TOTAL FOR THIS MONTH	FROM 1st DAY LAST MONTH	NEW TOTAL FROM 1st DAY
1.							
2.							
3.							
4.							
5.							
10.							
11.							
12.							
13.							
14.							
15.							

Photo

PHOTO

WEIGHT   _____
CHEST/BUST   _____
WAIST   _____
HIPS   _____

Goals For Next Month

_____
_____
_____
_____
_____
_____
_____
_____
_____
_____
_____
_____
_____
_____
_____
_____
_____
_____
_____
_____
_____
_____
_____
_____
_____
_____

Weekly Log

From: ___ / ___ / ___   To: ___ / ___ / ___

Body Weight — Beginning of Week _____   End of Week _____   Gain/Loss (+ or –) _____

NAME OF EXERCISE	SUN			MON			TUE			WED			THU			FRI			SAT		
	REPS	SETS	WT.	REPS	SETS	WT.	REPS	SETS	WT.	REPS	SETS	WT.	REPS	SETS	WT.	REPS	SETS	WT.	REPS	SETS	WT.
1.																					
2.																					
3.																					
4.																					
5.																					
6.																					
7.																					
8.																					
9.																					

AEROBICS	SUN TIME / DISTANCE	MON TIME / DISTANCE	TUE TIME / DISTANCE	WED TIME / DISTANCE	THU TIME / DISTANCE	FRI TIME / DISTANCE	SAT TIME / DISTANCE	TOTAL FOR WEEK
1.								
2.								
3.								
4.								
5.								
10.								
11.								
12.								
13.								
14.								
15.								

Weekly Log

Body Weight — Beginning of Week _____ End of Week _____ Gain/Loss (+ or –) _____

From: ___/___/___ To: ___/___/___

NAME OF EXERCISE	SUN			MON			TUE			WED			THU			FRI			SAT		
	REPS	SETS	WT.	REPS	SETS	WT.	REPS	SETS	WT.	REPS	SETS	WT.	REPS	SETS	WT.	REPS	SETS	WT.	REPS	SETS	WT.
1.																					
2.																					
3.																					
4.																					
5.																					
6.																					
7.																					
8.																					
9.																					

AEROBICS

	SUN TIME/DISTANCE	MON TIME/DISTANCE	TUE TIME/DISTANCE	WED TIME/DISTANCE	THU TIME/DISTANCE	FRI TIME/DISTANCE	SAT TIME/DISTANCE	TOTAL FOR WEEK
1.								
2.								
3.								
4.								
5.								
10.								
11.								
12.								
13.								
14.								
15.								

Weekly Log

From: ___ / ___ / ___   To: ___ / ___ / ___

Body Weight — Beginning of Week _____ End of Week _____ Gain/Loss (+ or –) _____

NAME OF EXERCISE	SUN			MON			TUE			WED			THU			FRI			SAT		
	REPS	SETS	WT.	REPS	SETS	WT.	REPS	SETS	WT.	REPS	SETS	WT.	REPS	SETS	WT.	REPS	SETS	WT.	REPS	SETS	WT.
1.																					
2.																					
3.																					
4.																					
5.																					
6.																					
7.																					
8.																					
9.																					

AEROBICS	SUN TIME / DISTANCE	MON TIME / DISTANCE	TUE TIME / DISTANCE	WED TIME / DISTANCE	THU TIME / DISTANCE	FRI TIME / DISTANCE	SAT TIME / DISTANCE	TOTAL FOR WEEK
1.								
2.								
3.								
4.								
5.								
10.								
11.								
12.								
13.								
14.								
15.								

Weekly Log

From: ___ / ___ / ___ To: ___ / ___ / ___

Body Weight — Beginning of Week _____ End of Week _____ Gain/Loss (+ or −) _____

NAME OF EXERCISE	SUN			MON			TUE			WED			THU			FRI			SAT		
	REPS	SETS	WT.	REPS	SETS	WT.	REPS	SETS	WT.	REPS	SETS	WT.	REPS	SETS	WT.	REPS	SETS	WT.	REPS	SETS	WT.
1.																					
2.																					
3.																					
4.																					
5.																					
6.																					
7.																					
8.																					
9.																					

AEROBICS	SUN TIME/DISTANCE	MON TIME/DISTANCE	TUE TIME/DISTANCE	WED TIME/DISTANCE	THU TIME/DISTANCE	FRI TIME/DISTANCE	SAT TIME/DISTANCE	TOTAL FOR WEEK
1.								
2.								
3.								
4.								
5.								
10.								
11.								
12.								
13.								
14.								
15.								

Notes and Comments

Notes and Comments

Four-Week Progress Chart

Body Weight — Beginning of Month _____ End of Month _____ Gain/Loss (+ or −) _____

3 MONTHLY

NAME OF EXERCISE	BEGINNING OF MONTH			END OF MONTH			GAIN/LOSS FOR MONTH						GAIN/LOSS FROM 1st DAY					
	REPS	SETS	WT.	REPS	SETS	WT.	+ OR −	REPS	+ OR −	SETS	+ OR −	WT.	+ OR −	REPS	+ OR −	SETS	+ OR −	WT.
1.																		
2.																		
3.																		
4.																		
5.																		
6.																		
7.																		
8.																		
9.																		

PROGRESS 3

AEROBICS	TOTAL FOR WEEK #1	TOTAL FOR WEEK #2	TOTAL FOR WEEK #3	TOTAL FOR WEEK #4	TOTAL FOR THIS MONTH	FROM 1st DAY LAST MONTH	NEW TOTAL FROM 1st DAY
1.							
2.							
3.							
4.							
5.							
10.							
11.							
12.							
13.							
14.							
15.							

Photo

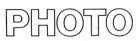

WEIGHT _____

CHEST/BUST _____

WAIST _____

HIPS _____

Goals For Next Month

_____
_____
_____
_____
_____
_____
_____
_____
_____
_____
_____
_____
_____
_____
_____
_____
_____
_____
_____
_____
_____
_____
_____
_____
_____
_____
_____

Weekly Log

Body Weight — Beginning of Week _____ End of Week _____

From: ___/___/___ To: ___/___/___ Gain/Loss (+ or –) _____

NAME OF EXERCISE	SUN			MON			TUE			WED			THU			FRI			SAT		
	REPS	SETS	WT.	REPS	SETS	WT.	REPS	SETS	WT.	REPS	SETS	WT.	REPS	SETS	WT.	REPS	SETS	WT.	REPS	SETS	WT.
1.																					
2.																					
3.																					
4.																					
5.																					
6.																					
7.																					
8.																					
9.																					

AEROBICS	SUN TIME / DISTANCE	MON TIME / DISTANCE	TUE TIME / DISTANCE	WED TIME / DISTANCE	THU TIME / DISTANCE	FRI TIME / DISTANCE	SAT TIME / DISTANCE	TOTAL FOR WEEK
10.								
11.								
12.								
13.								
14.								
15.								
1.								
2.								
3.								
4.								
5.								

73

Weekly Log

Body Weight — Beginning of Week _____ End of Week _____ From: __/__/__ To: __/__/__ Gain/Loss (+ or –) _____

NAME OF EXERCISE	SUN			MON			TUE			WED			THU			FRI			SAT		
	REPS	SETS	WT.	REPS	SETS	WT.	REPS	SETS	WT.	REPS	SETS	WT.	REPS	SETS	WT.	REPS	SETS	WT.	REPS	SETS	WT.
1.																					
2.																					
3.																					
4.																					
5.																					
6.																					
7.																					
8.																					
9.																					

AEROBICS

	SUN TIME / DISTANCE	MON TIME / DISTANCE	TUE TIME / DISTANCE	WED TIME / DISTANCE	THU TIME / DISTANCE	FRI TIME / DISTANCE	SAT TIME / DISTANCE	TOTAL FOR WEEK
1.								
2.								
3.								
4.								
5.								
10.								
11.								
12.								
13.								
14.								
15.								

Weekly Log

Body Weight — Beginning of Week _____ End of Week _____ Gain/Loss (+ or −)

From: ___ / ___ / ___ To: ___ / ___ / ___

NAME OF EXERCISE	SUN			MON			TUE			WED			THU			FRI			SAT		
	REPS	SETS	WT.	REPS	SETS	WT.	REPS	SETS	WT.	REPS	SETS	WT.	REPS	SETS	WT.	REPS	SETS	WT.	REPS	SETS	WT.
1.																					
2.																					
3.																					
4.																					
5.																					
6.																					
7.																					
8.																					
9.																					

AEROBICS

	SUN TIME/DISTANCE	MON TIME/DISTANCE	TUE TIME/DISTANCE	WED TIME/DISTANCE	THU TIME/DISTANCE	FRI TIME/DISTANCE	SAT TIME/DISTANCE	TOTAL FOR WEEK
1.								
2.								
3.								
4.								
5.								
10.								
11.								
12.								
13.								
14.								
15.								

Weekly Log

Body Weight — Beginning of Week _____ End of Week _____ Gain/Loss (+ or −) _____

From: ___/___/___ To: ___/___/___

NAME OF EXERCISE	SUN			MON			TUE			WED			THU			FRI			SAT		
	REPS	SETS	WT.	REPS	SETS	WT.	REPS	SETS	WT.	REPS	SETS	WT.	REPS	SETS	WT.	REPS	SETS	WT.	REPS	SETS	WT.
1.																					
2.																					
3.																					
4.																					
5.																					
6.																					
7.																					
8.																					
9.																					

AEROBICS	SUN TIME / DISTANCE	MON TIME / DISTANCE	TUE TIME / DISTANCE	WED TIME / DISTANCE	THU TIME / DISTANCE	FRI TIME / DISTANCE	SAT TIME / DISTANCE	TOTAL FOR WEEK
1.								
2.								
3.								
4.								
5.								
10.								
11.								
12.								
13.								
14.								
15.								

Notes and Comments

Notes and Comments

Four-Week Progress Chart

Body Weight — Beginning of Month _____ End of Month _____ From: __/__/__ To: __/__/__ Gain/Loss (+ or –) _____

NAME OF EXERCISE	BEGINNING OF MONTH			END OF MONTH			GAIN/LOSS FOR MONTH				GAIN/LOSS FROM 1st DAY			
	REPS	SETS	WT.	REPS	SETS	WT.	+ OR –	REPS	+ OR –	SETS	+ OR –	WT.	+ OR –	REPS	+ OR –	SETS	WT.
1.														
2.														
3.														
4.														
5.														
6.														
7.														
8.														
9.														

4 MONTHLY

PROGRESS 4

						NEW TOTAL FROM 1st DAY	FROM 1st DAY LAST MONTH	TOTAL FOR THIS MONTH	TOTAL FOR WEEK #4	TOTAL FOR WEEK #3	TOTAL FOR WEEK #2	TOTAL FOR WEEK #1	
10.													
11.													
12.													
13.													
14.													
15.													
AEROBICS													
1.													
2.													
3.													
4.													
5.													

Photo

PHOTO

WEIGHT   _____

CHEST/BUST   _____

WAIST   _____

HIPS   _____

Goals For Next Month

_____
_____
_____
_____
_____
_____
_____
_____
_____
_____
_____
_____
_____
_____
_____
_____
_____
_____
_____
_____
_____
_____
_____

Weekly Log

Body Weight — Beginning of Week _____ End of Week _____

From: ___/___/___ To: ___/___/___

Gain/Loss (+ or −) _____

NAME OF EXERCISE	SUN			MON			TUE			WED			THU			FRI			SAT		
	REPS	SETS	WT.	REPS	SETS	WT.	REPS	SETS	WT.	REPS	SETS	WT.	REPS	SETS	WT.	REPS	SETS	WT.	REPS	SETS	WT.
1.																					
2.																					
3.																					
4.																					
5.																					
6.																					
7.																					
8.																					
9.																					

AEROBICS	SUN. TIME/DISTANCE	MON. TIME/DISTANCE	TUE. TIME/DISTANCE	WED. TIME/DISTANCE	THU. TIME/DISTANCE	FRI. TIME/DISTANCE	SAT. TIME/DISTANCE	TOTAL FOR WEEK
1.								
2.								
3.								
4.								
5.								
10.								
11.								
12.								
13.								
14.								
15.								

Weekly Log

From: ___ / ___ / ___   To: ___ / ___ / ___

Body Weight — Beginning of Week _____ End of Week _____ Gain/Loss (+ or −) _____

NAME OF EXERCISE	SUN			MON			TUE			WED			THU			FRI			SAT		
	REPS	SETS	WT.	REPS	SETS	WT.	REPS	SETS	WT.	REPS	SETS	WT.	REPS	SETS	WT.	REPS	SETS	WT.	REPS	SETS	WT.
1.																					
2.																					
3.																					
4.																					
5.																					
6.																					
7.																					
8.																					
9.																					

	SUN TIME/DISTANCE	MON TIME/DISTANCE	TUE TIME/DISTANCE	WED TIME/DISTANCE	THU TIME/DISTANCE	FRI TIME/DISTANCE	SAT TIME/DISTANCE	TOTAL FOR WEEK
10.								
11.								
12.								
13.								
14.								
15.								

AEROBICS

	SUN TIME/DISTANCE	MON TIME/DISTANCE	TUE TIME/DISTANCE	WED TIME/DISTANCE	THU TIME/DISTANCE	FRI TIME/DISTANCE	SAT TIME/DISTANCE	TOTAL FOR WEEK
1.								
2.								
3.								
4.								
5.								

Weekly Log

Body Weight — Beginning of Week _____ End of Week _____ Gain/Loss (+ or –) _____

From: ___ / ___ / ___ To: ___ / ___ / ___

NAME OF EXERCISE	SUN			MON			TUE			WED			THU			FRI			SAT		
	REPS	SETS	WT.	REPS	SETS	WT.	REPS	SETS	WT.	REPS	SETS	WT.	REPS	SETS	WT.	REPS	SETS	WT.	REPS	SETS	WT.
1.																					
2.																					
3.																					
4.																					
5.																					
6.																					
7.																					
8.																					
9.																					

AEROBICS	SUN TIME/DISTANCE	MON TIME/DISTANCE	TUE TIME/DISTANCE	WED TIME/DISTANCE	THU TIME/DISTANCE	FRI TIME/DISTANCE	SAT TIME/DISTANCE	TOTAL FOR WEEK
1.								
2.								
3.								
4.								
5.								
10.								
11.								
12.								
13.								
14.								
15.								

Weekly Log

Body Weight — Beginning of Week _____ End of Week _____

From: ___ / ___ / ___   To: ___ / ___ / ___   Gain/Loss (+ or –) _____

NAME OF EXERCISE	SUN			MON			TUE			WED			THU			FRI			SAT		
	REPS	SETS	WT.	REPS	SETS	WT.	REPS	SETS	WT.	REPS	SETS	WT.	REPS	SETS	WT.	REPS	SETS	WT.	REPS	SETS	WT.
1.																					
2.																					
3.																					
4.																					
5.																					
6.																					
7.																					
8.																					
9.																					

AEROBICS	SUN TIME / DISTANCE	MON TIME / DISTANCE	TUE TIME / DISTANCE	WED TIME / DISTANCE	THU TIME / DISTANCE	FRI TIME / DISTANCE	SAT TIME / DISTANCE	TOTAL FOR WEEK
1.								
2.								
3.								
4.								
5.								
10.								
11.								
12.								
13.								
14.								
15.								

Notes and Comments

Notes and Comments

Four-Week Progress Chart

Body Weight — Beginning of Month _____ End of Month _____ From: __ / __ / __ To: __ / __ / __ Gain/Loss (+ or –)

5 MONTHLY

NAME OF EXERCISE	BEGINNING OF MONTH			END OF MONTH			GAIN/LOSS FOR MONTH				GAIN/LOSS FROM 1st DAY			
	REPS	SETS	WT.	REPS	SETS	WT.	+ OR – REPS	+ OR – SETS	+ OR –	WT.	+ OR – REPS	+ OR – SETS	+ OR –	WT.
1.														
2.														
3.														
4.														
5.														
6.														
7.														
8.														
9.														

PROGRESS 5

	TOTAL FOR WEEK #1	TOTAL FOR WEEK #2	TOTAL FOR WEEK #3	TOTAL FOR WEEK #4	TOTAL FOR THIS MONTH	FROM 1st DAY LAST MONTH	NEW TOTAL FROM 1st DAY
10.							
11.							
12.							
13.							
14.							
15.							
AEROBICS							
1.							
2.							
3.							
4.							
5.							

Photo

PHOTO

WEIGHT _____

CHEST/BUST _____

WAIST _____

HIPS _____

Goals For Next Month

Weekly Log

From: ___/___/___ To: ___/___/___

Body Weight — Beginning of Week _____ End of Week _____ Gain/Loss (+ or –) _____

NAME OF EXERCISE	SUN			MON			TUE			WED			THU			FRI			SAT		
	REPS	SETS	WT.	REPS	SETS	WT.	REPS	SETS	WT.	REPS	SETS	WT.	REPS	SETS	WT.	REPS	SETS	WT.	REPS	SETS	WT.
1.																					
2.																					
3.																					
4.																					
5.																					
6.																					
7.																					
8.																					
9.																					

AEROBICS	SUN TIME/DISTANCE	MON TIME/DISTANCE	TUE TIME/DISTANCE	WED TIME/DISTANCE	THU TIME/DISTANCE	FRI TIME/DISTANCE	SAT TIME/DISTANCE	TOTAL FOR WEEK
1.								
2.								
3.								
4.								
5.								
10.								
11.								
12.								
13.								
14.								
15.								

Weekly Log

Body Weight — Beginning of Week _____ End of Week _____ From: ___/___/___ To: ___/___/___

Gain/Loss (+ or −) _____

NAME OF EXERCISE	SUN			MON			TUE			WED			THU			FRI			SAT		
	REPS	SETS	WT.	REPS	SETS	WT.	REPS	SETS	WT.	REPS	SETS	WT.	REPS	SETS	WT.	REPS	SETS	WT.	REPS	SETS	WT.
1.																					
2.																					
3.																					
4.																					
5.																					
6.																					
7.																					
8.																					
9.																					

AEROBICS	SUN TIME/DISTANCE	MON TIME/DISTANCE	TUE TIME/DISTANCE	WED TIME/DISTANCE	THU TIME/DISTANCE	FRI TIME/DISTANCE	SAT TIME/DISTANCE	TOTAL FOR WEEK
1.								
2.								
3.								
4.								
5.								
10.								
11.								
12.								
13.								
14.								
15.								

Weekly Log

Body Weight — Beginning of Week _____ End of Week _____ From: ___ / ___ / ___ To: ___ / ___ / ___ Gain/Loss (+ or –) _____

NAME OF EXERCISE	SUN			MON			TUE			WED			THU			FRI			SAT		
	REPS	SETS	WT.	REPS	SETS	WT.	REPS	SETS	WT.	REPS	SETS	WT.	REPS	SETS	WT.	REPS	SETS	WT.	REPS	SETS	WT.
1.																					
2.																					
3.																					
4.																					
5.																					
6.																					
7.																					
8.																					
9.																					

AEROBICS

	SUN TIME / DISTANCE	MON TIME / DISTANCE	TUE TIME / DISTANCE	WED TIME / DISTANCE	THU TIME / DISTANCE	FRI TIME / DISTANCE	SAT TIME / DISTANCE	TOTAL FOR WEEK
1.								
2.								
3.								
4.								
5.								
10.								
11.								
12.								
13.								
14.								
15.								

Weekly Log

Body Weight — Beginning of Week _____ End of Week _____ From: ___ / ___ / ___ To: ___ / ___ / ___

Gain/Loss (+ or −) _____

NAME OF EXERCISE	SUN			MON			TUE			WED			THU			FRI			SAT		
	REPS	SETS	WT.	REPS	SETS	WT.	REPS	SETS	WT.	REPS	SETS	WT.	REPS	SETS	WT.	REPS	SETS	WT.	REPS	SETS	WT.
1.																					
2.																					
3.																					
4.																					
5.																					
6.																					
7.																					
8.																					
9.																					

AEROBICS	SUN TIME/DISTANCE	MON TIME/DISTANCE	TUE TIME/DISTANCE	WED TIME/DISTANCE	THU TIME/DISTANCE	FRI TIME/DISTANCE	SAT TIME/DISTANCE	TOTAL FOR WEEK
1.								
2.								
3.								
4.								
5.								
10.								
11.								
12.								
13.								
14.								
15.								

Notes and Comments

Notes and Comments

Four-Week Progress Chart

Body Weight — Beginning of Month _____ End of Month _____ From: __ / __ / __ To: __ / __ / __ Gain/Loss (+ or –) _____

6 MONTHLY

NAME OF EXERCISE	BEGINNING OF MONTH			END OF MONTH			GAIN/LOSS FOR MONTH				GAIN/LOSS FROM 1st DAY			
	REPS	SETS	WT.	REPS	SETS	WT.	+ OR –	REPS	+ OR –	SETS	+ OR –	WT.	+ OR –	REPS	+ OR –	SETS	+ OR –	WT.
1.															
2.															
3.															
4.															
5.															
6.															
7.															
8.															
9.															

PROGRESS 6

AEROBICS	TOTAL FOR WEEK #1	TOTAL FOR WEEK #2	TOTAL FOR WEEK #3	TOTAL FOR WEEK #4	TOTAL FOR THIS MONTH	FROM 1st DAY LAST MONTH	NEW TOTAL FROM 1st DAY
1.							
2.							
3.							
4.							
5.							
10.							
11.							
12.							
13.							
14.							
15.							

Goals For Next Month

_____
_____
_____
_____
_____
_____
_____
_____
_____
_____
_____
_____
_____
_____
_____
_____
_____
_____
_____
_____
_____
_____
_____
_____

Six Month Summary

WEIGHT & MEASUREMENTS

END OF MONTH INFORMATION	1st MONTH	2nd MONTH	3rd MONTH	4th MONTH	5th MONTH	6th MONTH		
	MONTH	MONTH	MONTH	MONTH	MONTH	MONTH	GAIN/LOSS	
MEASUREMENT	YEAR	YEAR	YEAR	YEAR	YEAR	YEAR	+ OR −	
HEIGHT								
WEIGHT								
CHEST / BUST								
WAIST								
HIPS								
NECK								
SHOULDERS								
RIGHT BICEPS								
LEFT BICEPS								
RIGHT FOREARM								
LEFT FOREARM								
WRISTS								
RIGHT THIGH								
LEFT THIGH								
RIGHT CALF								
LEFT CALF								
ANKLES								

Six Month Summary

STRENGTH
(WEIGHT TRAINING)

END OF MONTH INFORMATION	1st MONTH	2nd MONTH	3rd MONTH	4th MONTH	5th MONTH	6th MONTH		
NAME OF EXERCISE	MONTH / YEAR	MONTH / YEAR	MONTH / YEAR	MONTH / YEAR	MONTH / YEAR	MONTH / YEAR	**GAIN/LOSS** + OR –	
1.								
2.								
3.								
4.								
5.								
6.								
7.								
8.								
9.								
10.								
11.								
12.								
13.								
14.								
15.								
16.								
17.								
18.								
19.								
20.								
21.								

Six Month Summary

ENDURANCE
(AEROBICS)

END OF MONTH INFORMATION	1st MONTH	2nd MONTH	3rd MONTH	4th MONTH	5th MONTH	6th MONTH	
NAME OF EXERCISE	MONTH / YEAR	MONTH / YEAR	MONTH / YEAR	MONTH / YEAR	MONTH / YEAR	MONTH / YEAR	**GAIN/LOSS** + OR −
1.							
2.							
3.							
4.							
5.							
6.							
7.							
8.							
9.							
10.							
11.							
12.							
13.							
14.							
15.							
16.							
17.							

CARDIOVASCULAR FITNESS

PULSE RATE							
BLOOD PRESSURE							
PULSE RECOVERY RATE							

Goals for Next Six Months

Goals for Next Six Months

_____

_____

_____

_____

_____

_____

_____

_____

_____

_____

_____

_____

_____

_____

_____

_____

_____

_____

_____

_____

_____

_____

_____

_____

_____

_____

_____

Notes

Notes

Notes

Notes